First Aid for Kids

Know What To Do

To Help Your Child

I0450160

Health Learning Series

M. Usman

Mendon Cottage Books

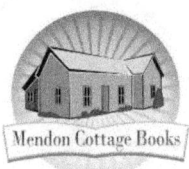

JD-Biz Publishing

All Rights Reserved.

No part of this publication may be reproduced in any form or by any means, including scanning, photocopying, or otherwise without prior written permission from JD-Biz Corp Copyright © 2014

All Images Licensed by Fotolia and 123RF.

Disclaimer

The information is this book is provided for informational purposes only. It is not intended to be used and medical advice or a substitute for proper medical treatment by a qualified health care provider. The information is believed to be accurate as presented based on research by the author.

The contents have not been evaluated by the U.S. Food and Drug Administration or any other Government or Health Organization and the contents in this book are not to be used to treat cure or prevent disease.

The author or publisher is not responsible for the use or safety of any diet, procedure or treatment mentioned in this book. The author or publisher is not responsible for errors or omissions that may exist.

Warning

The Book is for informational purposes only and before taking on any diet, treatment or medical procedure, it is recommended to consult with your primary health care provider.

Our books are available at

1. Amazon.com
2. Barnes and Noble
3. Itunes
4. Kobo
5. Smashwords
6. Google Play Books

Table of Contents

Introduction

Raising or bringing up children is a very tough job for the parents. Every parent would do anything to keep their children away from all harms and injuries. You might try to be like a protective shield for your child all the time, but sometimes it becomes impossible for you to guard your kids against the odds. Your little champions cannot afford to stay in one place. Children are naturally intrigued by every object they come across. It's their intrinsic ability to explore everything. The curiosity that dwells inside them makes them kind of restless (we've all been kids so it's understandable). No matter how many times you forbid your kids from doing dangerous activities or touching harmful things, they simply won't stop doing it. You can't keep an eye on your kids all day, can you? Once they're out of your sight, they might up end up in some danger. What would you do if your baby (God forbid) or someone else's baby starts choking after having ingested a coin? What would you do to save that baby? Do you think you're prepared to cope with that emergency? If not, then you need not worry. This book is all you need to keep your baby safe in any emergency.

This book is a complete guide for you that can help you manage any emergency situation that you and your baby might face. Calling for emergency help is certainly the first thing to do, but you can't wait for help and stand there and do nothing. After reading this book, you'll be equipped with different techniques and maneuvers that are simple, yet effective, and can prove to be the difference between your baby's safety and danger. We don't mean to startle you, but being prepared is always better than being sorry. So take a deep breath here and start with us on your journey to become an even better mother/father to your children.

Chapter 1 – First Aid for Choking

Children are always willing to put anything into their mouths and can easily choke as well. Even I choked once in my childhood after I ingested a coin. When a foreign body lodges into the windpipe, it results in choking or obstruction of the airway. Once the airway gets blocked, the air can't find its way to the lungs. Like an engine needs fuel to run, the vital organs of the body require an uninterrupted supply of oxygen for their survival. Cutting off oxygen to the tissues can lead to their death. For instance, the brain can't survive the shortage of oxygen for more than 4-5 minutes. This explains how life threatening choking can be.

So, if your child accidently comes across a choking emergency, you must be already prepared to deal with it. This can be made possible only if you are equipped with the sufficient knowledge of basic first aid techniques for choking. Here are some danger signs that can tell you that your child is choking:

- Gasping and wheezing
- Inability to talk
- Clenching the throat with fingers
- Coughing
- Turning blue of the lips and face

If you suddenly see any of the above danger signs, it's time be alarmed and to come into action quickly, without wasting a single moment. The more time you waste panicking, the more danger you will put your child into.

First Aid for Choking in Babies or Infants (less than 1 year of age)

- **Back blows:** If you see your child choking, do not waste a single second. Pick your child up and start giving him back blows immediately. This is the simplest thing you can try at home to help your choking child. First hold the baby in a face down position and support him along your thigh. Keep the head of baby lower than the level of the rest of the body. This way the gravity will force the foreign body to come out of the windpipe easily. Now, with the heel of your hand, firmly hit the baby's back at the point midway between the two shoulder blades. Keep giving blows until the foreign object dislodges.

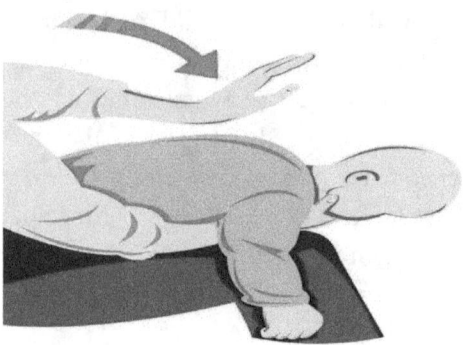

- **Chest thrusts:** When the back blows fail to dislodge the obstructing object, then chest thrusts become the next hope for relieving the choking. Turn the baby over and hold him in your lap. Place the two fingers of the other hand, in the middle of breastbone of the baby, just below the nipples. Press the chest upward and inward five times. Pushes must not be too hard as it can fracture the baby's ribs. Don't forget to check baby's mouth after each cycle of back blows and chest thrusts. If you are able to see the foreign body, try to remove it by doing finger sweep. Slowly insert the index finger of your hand into the mouth of the baby along his cheek. Make a hook of your finger and scoop out the obstructing object with it. If the object does not come out, immediately call 911 or a rescue center and continue doing back blows and chest thrust alternatively, until the rescue team arrives.

First Aid for Choking in Children (above the age of 1 year)

If the child is coughing or trying to speak, don't do anything. Just encourage your child to cough and expel out the foreign object. But, if the object does not come out and your child now is even unable to speak then give back blows and do abdominal thrusts.

- **Back blows:** Make the child lean forward slightly. Support him by placing your one hand on his chest. Now, with the heel of other hand give sharp back blows between the two shoulder blades. Give five back blows until the obstruction is relieved. But, if the child continues to choke, go for the abdominal thrusts.

- **Abdominal thrusts (Heimlich manuever):** Like back blows, abdominal thrusts are very simple and easy to do. All you need to know is the correct technique of doing them. Ask the child (or make him) slightly bend or lean forward. Wrap your arms around his waist and clench your one hand and place it at the midpoint between the navel and the tip of the breast bone. Now, grasp this fist with the help of other hand and give pushes inward and upward. Repeat it five times. If the obstruction persists, call 911 or a first aid center and continue doing alternative cycles of back blows and abdominal thrust until the help arrives. But, if the child becomes unconscious, stop doing back blows and abdominal thrusts. Look for breathing and start doing cardiopulmonary resuscitation (CPR) as soon as possible.

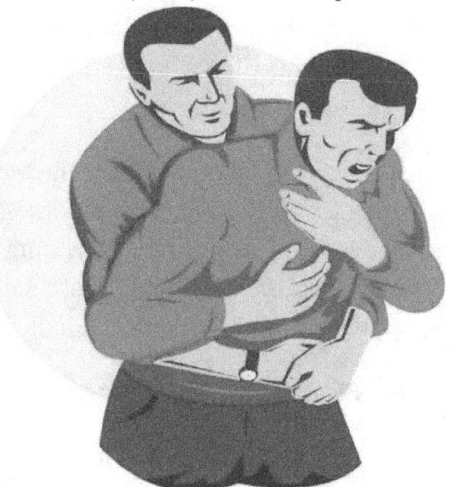

Chapter 2 – Cardiopulmonary Resuscitation (CPR)

CPR stands for cardiopulmonary resuscitation. The CPR technique serves the purpose of a lifesaving tool when all other strategies fail to rescue the baby's life. Cardiopulmonary resuscitation is applicable only when the victim is unconscious and is not breathing. This state of altered consciousness happens when the heart comes to arrest or breathing stops suddenly as seen in emergency situations like drowning, suffocation, choking, electric shock, poisoning, and head injuries. Children are more likely to become the victims of such situations. You might have heard or read news stories or seen on TV news channels that a mother left her child, for a moment, in the bathtub and in the next few moments the child was found dead due to drowning. Unfortunately, such incidences of drowning and choking are getting very common in children. Even your minor negligence can cost your child his life. Whatever the circumstances you face, you must know how to deal with it.

If you come across an emergency situation where the baby is unconscious and is not breathing, then start CPR as soon as possible. You can well imagine what would happen if the heart or the breathing stops suddenly. The objective of CPR is to kick start the heart and to rescue the breathing, so that the blood supply and oxygenation of tissue is maintained.

Here are the steps to do CPR in the correct way:

- First, assess the baby for responsiveness. Tap on the feet or the shoulders of the baby. If he does not respond, place him on his back carefully on a flat surface (Doing CPR on a mattress would never help).
- Look for the signs of breathing like chest movements and breathing sounds. Bring your cheek near to the baby's nostrils to feel his breath or try to hear it.
- If the baby is not responding or breathing, shout for help or call 911 or a rescue center for immediate help.
- Now, tilt the baby's head back by applying gentle pressure on his forehead. Put the two fingers of the other hand on the bony protuberance of the chin and then lift the chin up. Doing this will help in keeping the airway patent by keeping the tongue from falling fall back and

obstructing the airway. Avoid tilting the head too much. Pay special attention if the child has any head or spinal injuries, in such cases, tilting the head should be avoided as it can further aggravate the injury.

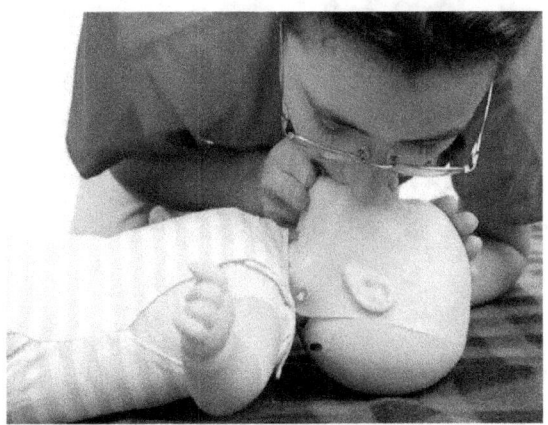

- Pinch the baby's nostrils with the hand placed on his forehead. Take a deep breath and seal your mouth around the baby's mouth tightly. Blow the air gently into his mouth. In the meantime, keep looking at the chest of the baby for a chest rise. When the chest rises, stop for a few seconds, letting the air flow out and continuing to the next breath. Give two rescue breaths in this way.
- Now, place two fingers in the center of the baby's chest slightly below the nipple line. Compress the chest down about 1 to 1 ½ inches. For children older than 1 year, you can use the heel of one hand to do the chest compressions. Give 100 compressions per minutes. After every 30 compressions, give two rescue breaths and continue the cycle of chest compression and rescue breaths until the help arrives. Do not push too hard as the child's delicate ribs are more prone to fractures.

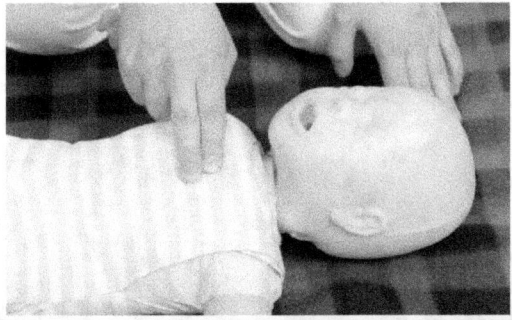

- After 5 cycles, check for carotid pulse. If you can feel the pulse then stop. Otherwise keep doing CPR (for hours if you have to) until the help arrives.

Chapter 3 - First Aid for Fractures and Sprains

Fractures and sprains are something faced very often by children. You cannot expect your child to sit quietly in one place. Young children are energetic and enthusiastic, playing and jumping here and there. It would not be wrong to say that children are fearless. Your heart may skip a beat while watching your child jump off the bed or sofa recklessly, but your child won't even bother to think about the consequences he can suffer from after falling. Children's bones are soft and not mature enough to withstand the impact of falling. That is why; they are more prone to injuries and fractures.

If your child falls and gets a fracture, do not get panic. Try to stay calm and concentrate on how you can give your child the immediate care or first aid. The injured area will be reddened, swollen, bruised and extremely painful. Well, fractures and sprains are, sometimes, difficult to be differentiated on the basis of their appearance and symptoms. Therefore, the first aid for both fractures and sprains is a bit similar.

First Aid for Fractures

- If you suspect that your child has a broken or fractured bone, first carefully observe the injured area. Look for bleeding. If there is bleeding, take a clean cloth and use it to apply gentle pressure on the bleeding area. After applying pressure, wrap a sterile dressing around the wound, loosely.
- The only way to manage the fractured bone is by immobilizing the affected part of the limb. Do not let your child move, as moving the fractured part can lead to further swelling, pain and many other complications. Encourage the child to stay calm and to avoid unnecessary movement, as much as possible.
- If the limb bone is fractured, you can place a pillow under the limb to make the child more comfortable. This will help in restricting the limb movement as well.
- Never ever try to realign or straighten the fractured bones, as in doing so, you can cause further damage.
- Take a few ice cubes, wrap them in a cloth and apply this ice pack to the affected area for 10 - 15 minutes. The cooling effect of the ice pack will reduce the swelling and will help diminish the pain.

- Applying hot compresses is the biggest mistake. Never use hot compresses or massage on the affected area because it promotes swelling.
- You can make use of splints to immobilize the fractured limb, if necessary. Splints can be made easily by using things like newspapers, magazines, cardboard, or a piece of cloth. Roll up a newspaper or magazine and wrap it around the broken bone. Tie the splints with a belt, tape, or a piece of cloth. Splints should not be tied too tight because it can cut off the blood circulation to the affected area. If splinting the broken bone causes inconvenience or pain to the child, it's better to remove the splints. You may wrap the splints in a cloth or soft towel to cushion the fractured bone from the impact of splint.
- For the fractures of the arm and forearm, a sling can be used to immobilize the fractured limb. Take a square shaped cloth, like a pillow case, and fold it to form a triangle. Carefully place the child's forearm in the sling. Pull the ends of the slings until the elbow comes to the level of the chest. Finally, tie the edges of the sling around the side of the neck of the child.
- If you feel that the child's condition is serious or there is a fracture of the head, ribs and pelvis, call an ambulance immediately, or take the child to the hospital to seek proper medical help (even if the fracture is minor).

First Aid for Sprains and Strains:

When the muscles or ligaments are overstretched or torn, it is termed as a sprain or strain. A sprain is different from a fractured bone, but the symptoms of both are the same like pain, redness, and swelling. But, the pain associated with a sprain is less severe when compared to the fractures. Just remember one word, **RICE**, as a first aid for sprains and strains. The word RICE stands **for rest, ice, compression and elevation**. So, whenever your child gets a twisted ankle, just recall this word and you will be able to help your child on your own.

- **Rest:** Rest is the best thing that can help your child. Immobilizing the affected limb is the only way to let the child recover. It's pretty hard for your child to just stay in one place, but as a responsible parent, you will have to keep an eye on him to make sure that the he does not move his limb unnecessarily. Taking rest for 1-2 days will make him feel much better.

- **Ice:** Apply an ice pack on the affected area. Never apply ice directly to the skin. Always wrap it in a cloth or towel, and then use it to compress the affected site gently. Ice packs are amazingly helpful in reducing the pain and swelling. These cold compresses can be applied every few hours.

- **Compression:** When a sprain occurs, the blood vessels in that area become a bit leaky. The blood fluid leaks out from the vessels into the surrounding tissue, where it accumulates and leads to swelling. The easiest way to reduce the swelling is to wrap the injured area with a bandage, firmly. You can also make your child wear an elastic bandage instead of a regular bandage. The bandage helps in reducing the swelling by compressing the vessels.

- **Elevation:** The last component of RICE therapy is elevation. Keep the injured area slightly elevated by placing a pillow beneath it. Elevating the limb minimizes the blood flow to the affected area (without compromising the blood supply) and reduces swelling.

Chapter 4 - First Aid for Nosebleeds

Do you get scared when you see blood dripping from your child's nose? Well, there is nothing to be worried about if your child gets a nosebleed once in a while. A nosebleed, generally, is not considered a serious or emergency condition. It is a self-limiting condition that can be well managed at home just by following a few first aid tips. Nosebleeds are very common in children, especially in children aged 3-10 years. The nasal septum, the partition separating the two nostrils from each other, is the area of rich blood supply. Here, the blood vessels are fragile and are covered by a thin layer of tissue or membrane. Being so exposed and fragile makes these vessels more prone to bursting. When one of these vessels bursts, it leads to bleeding from the nose. Therefore, nose picking is one the most common causes of nose bleeding or epistaxis. The other causes of nose bleeds include injury, infections, allergies, boils, and dryness of the nose, foreign body and bleeding or clotting disorders.

Here is a simple way to control the nose bleeding within minutes at home:

- Keep your child calm. Running at the sight of blood can actually make the bleeding worse.
- Make your child sit down, comfortably, in an upright position. Make him lean forward. If the child leans back, there is the possibility he may swallow the blood. Swallowing the blood may induce vomiting, which might end up in aggravating the bleeding.
- Now, using your thumb and index finger, gently pinch the lower or soft part of the nose. Continue pinching the nostrils for at least 10 minutes. Applying pressure to the nose will compress the leaking vessel and will trigger clot formation. If you do not do it properly for 10 minutes, the bleeding may start again, because 10 minutes is the approximate time for the clot to form. If you keep on checking every minute whether the bleeding has stopped or not, the bleeding may not stop because you've not given enough time for the blood to clot.
- In the meanwhile, encourage the child to breath from the mouth. Applying an ice pack on the nose, while keeping the nose pinched, may be helpful in reducing the blood loss.
- Release the pressure after 10 minutes. If the bleeding still continues, again pinch the nose for 5-10 minutes.

- But if the bleeding resists stopping, immediately seek emergency medical help.
- If the nose bleeding occurs after an injury, trauma or accident, it should be considered as a medical emergency.

How to avoid nose bleeding in children?

By following a few simple instructions and precautionary measures, the incidences of nose bleeding in the children can be minimized:

- Tell your child not to blow or pick his nose for a whole day after bleeding.
- Discourage the habit of nose picking in children as it is the predominant cause of nose bleeding in children.
- Children are more prone to get nose bleeds in dry climates and winters. To avoid the dryness of the nose, keep it moist by using humidifiers and saline nasal sprays. You may apply a bit of petroleum jelly (Vaseline) in the nose to retain its moisture.
- If your child is having a runny nose all the time along with episodic nose bleeds, this may be due to a nose allergy or infection. In such cases, the nose bleeding gets cured on its own when the underlying medical cause is treated.

Chapter 5 - First Aid for Electric Shock

Things like electric wires, switch boards, and electric appliances are especially fascinating for your little kiddo. Whenever you see your kid plugging his fingers in the switch board or biting an electric wire, it scares you, so you rush towards your child to pull him away from the electric source. But what if you are busy somewhere and your child is experimenting with electric wires? Obviously, the outcomes of this can be very dangerous.

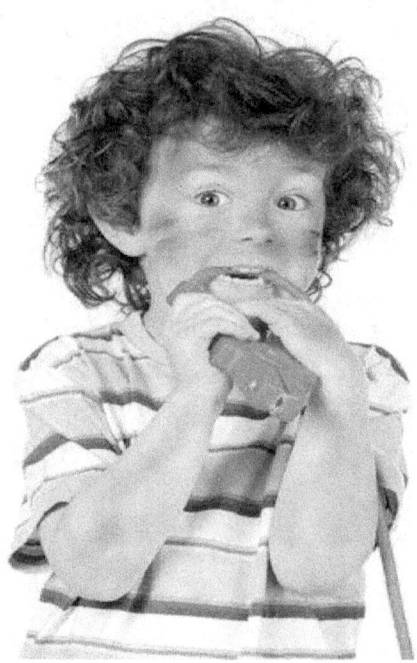

The human body is a good conductor of electric current so it is possible that your child may get an electric injury or electric shock. The manifestations of electric shock vary from discomfort and minor burns to severe skin burns, numbness, altered consciousness, seizures, muscle contractions, breathing difficulty, irregular heartbeats, and cardiac arrest. The outcomes of electrical current injury depend on the strength of electric current and duration of contact with the current source. Low voltage current may produce just minor burns while high voltage current can lead to fatal consequences.

Unfortunately, if such a thing happens, you must be the first one to save your child on the spot. Here is the way to rescue your child from electric shock:

- Turn off the electric source. Unplug the cord as soon as possible. Be careful since you are also exposed to the same risk of getting electric current while doing this. Use some type of non-conducting material, like wooden sticks, rolled up magazines, or newspapers, to handle with the electric current source.
- If the situation is serious, call the emergency number like 911.
- Do not try to touch the child when he is in contact with the electric current, because in doing so the current can pass through your body as well. If it is not possible for you to switch off the electric supply, quickly pull away the child from source of current. But, the precaution here is the same as above. Use non-conducting material such as a blanket, rubber items, newspaper, a door mat or wooden stick to separate the child from the source. Never use metallic object as metals are excellent conductors of electricity.
- Make sure the place you are standing, while rescuing the child, is completely dry. If you are barefoot, stand on something, a door mat or a piece of newspaper.
- Once you pull the child away from the source, check for breathing. If the child is unconscious and is not breathing, start CPR immediately.
- If the child becomes pale and feels cold and clammy, it means he is in a state of shock. Elevate the child's legs and wrap him in a blanket. Keep him warm as much as possible. Take the child to the hospital emergency room or call the local emergency rescue teams.
- If the child is fine and just has minor skin burns, give him the first aid for burns. Carefully wash the burn with cool water and wrap it with a sterile dressing. Do consult a doctor afterward to make sure the child is completely fine.

How can you prevent electric shock in children?

- Make sure that all electrical wires are properly insulated.
- Do not let your child handle electrical devices.
- If possible, do not use electrical devices, like irons, in the presence of children or unplug them as soon as you finish using them.

- Toys that are electrically operated must not be given to the children, especially when they are at the age of 3-5 years.
- You can use child safety plugs or safety covers to reduce the risk of electrical injuries in children.
- Do not allow your child to touch electrical cords.
- For older children, you must teach them about the hazards of electric current.

Chapter 6 - First Aid for Accidental Poisoning

"Keep out of reach of children". You might have read this phrase several times on the precautionary label of medicines, chemical bottles, pesticides, household detergents and cleaners. Never underestimate a child's exploring nature. You won't think of this even in your wildest dreams, but your child can approach the hidden nooks of your home where you store such things, thinking they might be safe there. Accidental poisoning can be of various forms. The child can either ingest the poison while trying to taste it or drop it on his skin.

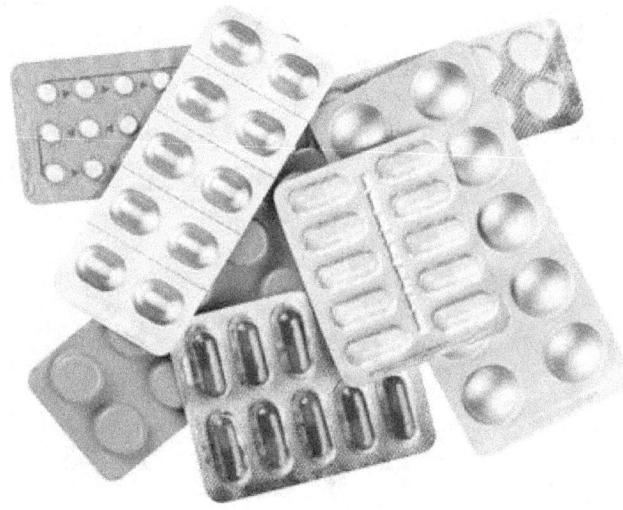

Some chemicals produce poisonous fumes, so the poison can be inhaled too. The symptoms of poisoning include vomiting, burns around the mouth, difficulty in breathing, drowsiness and seizures. The intensity of poisoning depends on the type of poison and the way it enters the child's body.

If you suspect your child has been poisoned, take the following measures immediately to save the child from serious outcomes.

- Call the nearby poison control center without wasting a single moment.

- If poison comes in contact with the skin, remove the clothing from the affected area and rinse it with lukewarm water for 15-20 minutes. Seek medical help afterwards.
- If the child inhales the poison, move him away from the suffocating environment. Bring him in fresh air immediately.
- If you suspect the child has ingested the poison, first look at the poison he swallowed. You may find an empty poison bottle nearby. Household detergents, cleansers, and drugs are the main culprits of accidental poisoning in kids. Look into the child's mouth. If you see any poisonous material, take it out with a finger. Make sure not to induce vomiting because vomiting can worsen the child's condition.
- If the child becomes unconscious and has difficulty in breathing, start doing CPR and give rescue breaths. If you see the poison around the lips and mouth, wash it before giving rescue breaths. Continue doing CPR until the help arrives.
- By any chance, if the child splashes poison into his eyes, then hold him tightly and flush his eyes with water for 15 minutes. Then take him to the doctor for further management.

Chapter 7 - First Aid for Vomiting and Diarrhea

Children and babies suffer from vomiting and diarrhea every now and then. The reasons for diarrhea in children can be a gut infection, inability to digest food properly, poor hygiene, eating contaminated food, and so on. But, more often, the culprit for diarrhea in babies is their immature gut. A baby's gut becomes mature with time. A baby cannot digest everything given to him, especially lactose containing products. Therefore, diarrhea, due to lactose intolerance, is highly common in babies.

But when would you say that your child is suffering from diarrhea? According to the world health organization criteria if the child passes 3 loose stools per day it means he is having diarrhea. Every mother must be guided about the first aid tips for diarrhea, so they can prevent their children from getting dehydrated. Here is the first aid plan for dealing with diarrhea in children.

- Give plenty of boiled water and fresh juices to the child (if the child is more than 2 years of age). Continuing fluid therapy is the only way for keeping the child well hydrated. Do not gives sodas or caffeine drinks.
- You can also give hydration solutions like Pedialyte or ORS to babies. Give a few sips of ORS to the child after he passes stool. This will help in compensating for the water and electrolyte loss.
- If the mother is breastfeeding the child, she must continue feeding him, because mother's milk is the best therapy for babies, since it contains all the essential components along with antibodies that will help the child in his fight against the infections.
- Give your child semi solid and easily digestible foods like mashed banana, rice or toast (if the child has reached the age of weaning).
- If the child shows danger signs like drowsiness, sunken eyes, dry mouth, fever or bloody diarrhea, immediately take him to the hospital.

Chapter 8 – First Aid for Fever

Fever is not a disease, but shows that your baby's insides are not functioning well. When the body temperature rises above the normal level, it is said to be a fever. Do not worry if your child gets fever, because most of the time it resolves on its own without needing any medical help. The causes of fever in children include sore throat, chest infections, ear infections, common cold, flu, teething, and vaccinations.

If the doctor is not available at that time, you can give first aid to your child at home to reduce his fever:

- First check the temperature using a thermometer. Don't put it in the baby's mouth. Use the armpit for that purpose.
- Give your child the child based formula of acetaminophen or ibuprofen. The doses must be given correctly as per instructed on the label. Never give aspirin to the children as it can cause Reye syndrome in them.
- If the child is overdressed, remove extra clothing. Leave only the single layer of clothing and wrap the child in a thin blanket sheet.
- Sponging the face, legs and arms with a wet cloth dipped in water can help in bringing down the fever.
- Give plenty of fluids, fresh juices and soups to the child. Avoid giving caffeinated drinks.
- Contact the doctor if the child becomes drowsy or the fever does not ward off. If the baby less than 3 months of age has a fever of 100.4 degrees Fahrenheit or the baby is less than 6 months of age and has a fever of 102.2 Fahrenheit, consider it serious.

Chapter 9 - First Aid for Bleeding or Wounds

What would you do if your child jumps off the sofa recklessly and comes to you with a bleeding wound on his forehead? Here are some simple steps to follow:

- First wash your hands and dry them.
- Wash the wound with a plenty of water for 15-20 seconds to remove the dirt and germs from the wound.
- If the wound is bleeding, apply pressure on the wound with gauze for 5-10 minutes until the bleeding stops.
- Once the bleeding stops, apply an antibiotic cream on the wound and cover it with a sterile bandage.
- If the child is bleeding heavily, take a clean cloth or a dressing and apply pressure on the bleeding point with it.
- For the injuries of the limbs, raise the injured limb to reduce the blood flow to the affected area.
- Wrap the bleeding area firmly with a sterile dressing. If the dressing soaks the blood, wrap more dressings around it.
- Keep applying pressure on the bleeding area until you seek emergency medical help.
- If the bleeding continues, go to a hospital or call 911.

Chapter 10 - First Aid for Burns

Burns can be of various types like chemical burns, electrical burns, flame burns and hot liquid burns. Whatever the type of the burn might be the management for all the burn is more or less same. Superficial burns can be managed well at home while deep burns need emergency medical attention. First aid for burns includes the following steps:

- Cool the burned area first by putting it under cold running water for 15-20 min.
- After cooling the burn, let it dry and wrap it with a sterile dressing.
- Give analgesics like acetaminophen or ibuprofen to the child.
- Do not apply ice, butter or any ointment on the burn.
- For the deep burns or burn with bleeding, it is suggested to leave the clothing that sticks to the burned area. Do not immerse the burned part in water. Take a wet cloth and pat the burned area with it. Raise the affected part above the level of the heart to prevent fluid loss and dehydration.
- Cover the burned area with sterile dressing and take the child immediately to the hospital emergency or call the local emergency number.
- If the child becomes unconscious and stops breathing, start doing CPR till the help arrives.

Chapter 11 - First aid for allergy

Allergies can occur due to many reasons like food, dust, insect bites and stings. The symptoms of allergies are redness and blotching of the skin, tingling sensations, severe itching, skin rashes, runny eyes and watery nose.

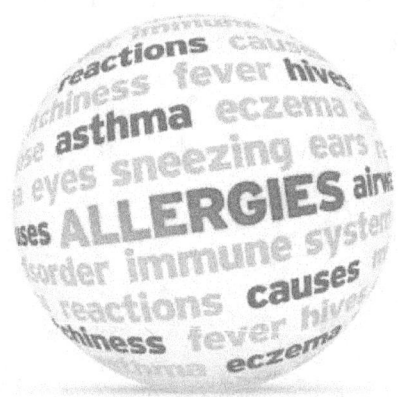

Allergic reactions can be looked after at home by using the following first aid tips:

- For mild allergy symptoms like skin rashes and itching, give the child over the counter anti-allergy or antihistamine medicine.
- Applying ice packs to the affected area can reduce the swelling and itching.
- If the child shows symptoms of anaphylactic shock, such as dizziness, chest tightness or swelling of the tongue, call for help or take the child to the hospital.
- Start CPR if the child becomes unresponsive. Do it until the help arrives.

Conclusion

You can never be prepared for every situation. Life moves fast and some situations arise before you even blink your eyes. We have covered several different categories in this book, which I hope have taught you a few things. Read this book over and over until you are able to memorize how to handle each situation, like it is second nature to you. This book is meant to teach the basics of first aid for several different circumstances, so keep practicing! And remember, be safe!

Author Bio

Muhammad Usman is a distinguished medical graduate of Allama Iqbal medical college (AIMC). He is a professional writer who has been in the field for more than 4 years. During this time he has produced 10,000+ articles, blogs and eBooks on various niches related to diseases, health, fitness, nutrition and well-being. He is a regular contributor to several journals related to medicine and surgery. He is the editor of several journals and newspapers.

Check out some of the other JD-Biz Publishing books
Gardening Series on Amazon

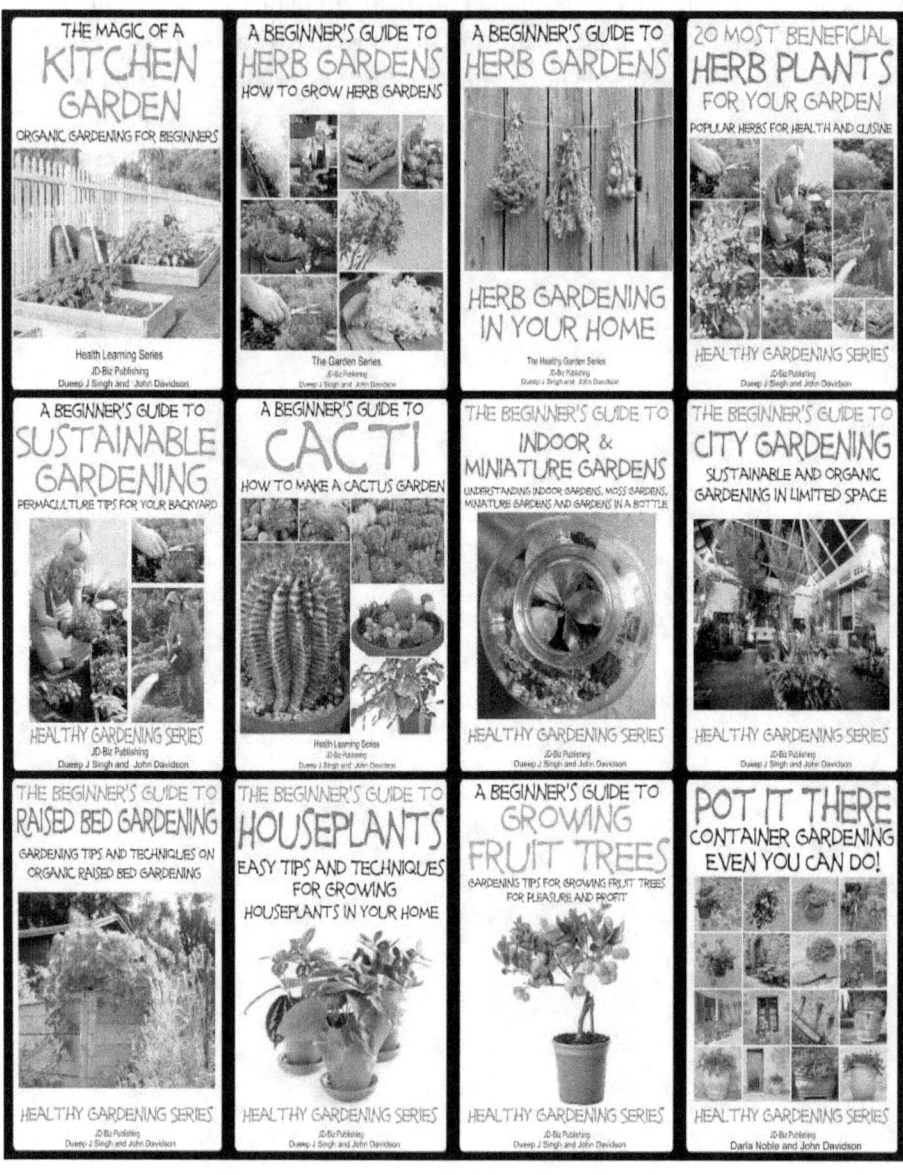

Health Learning Series

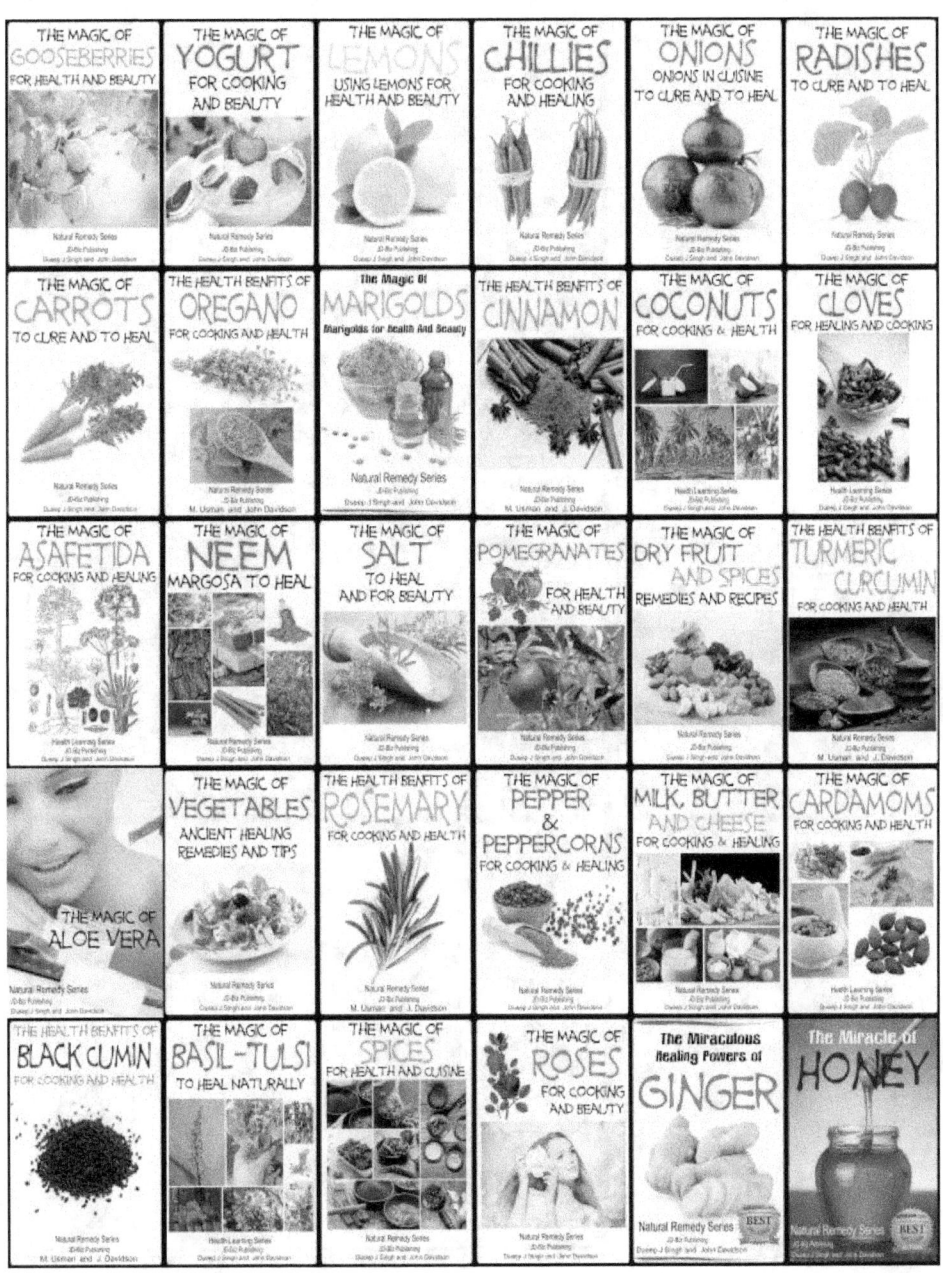

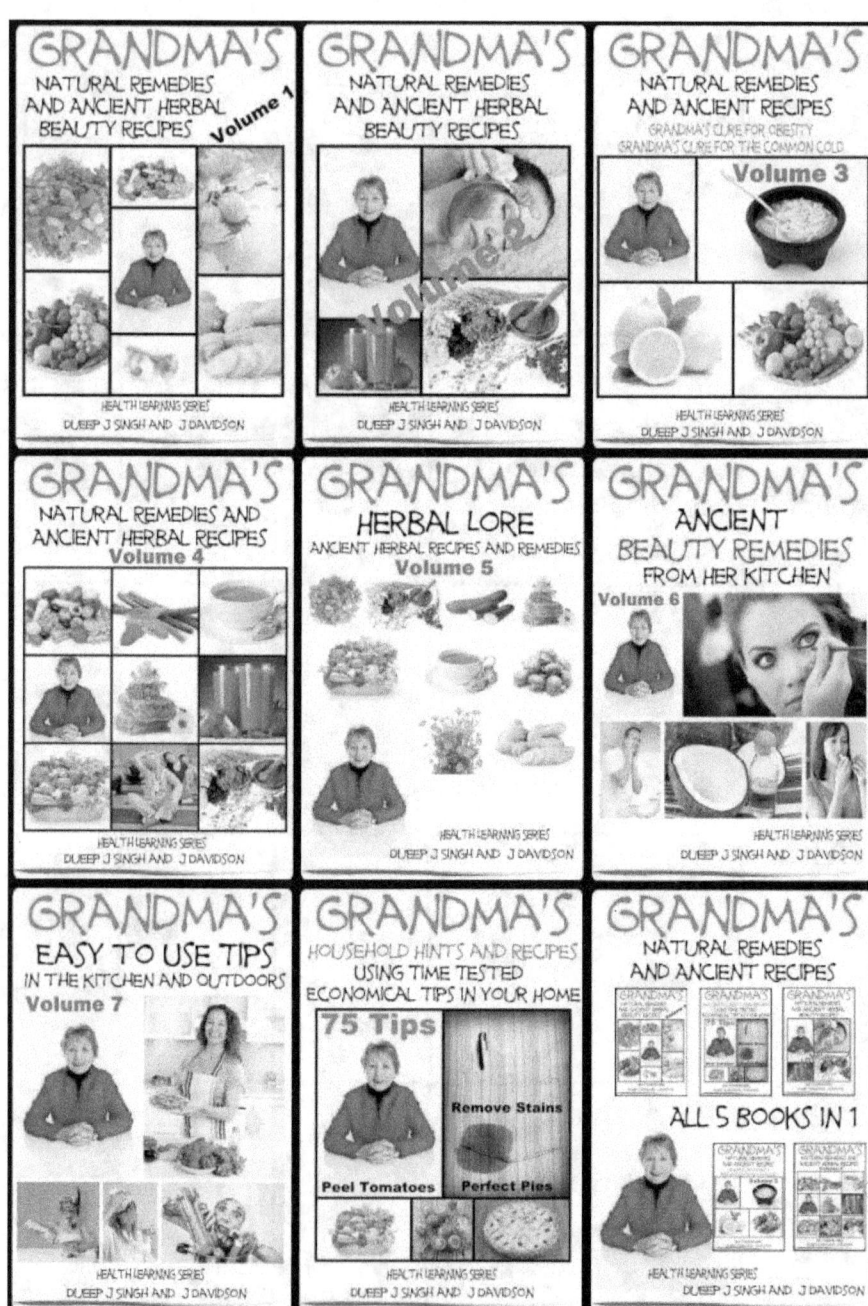

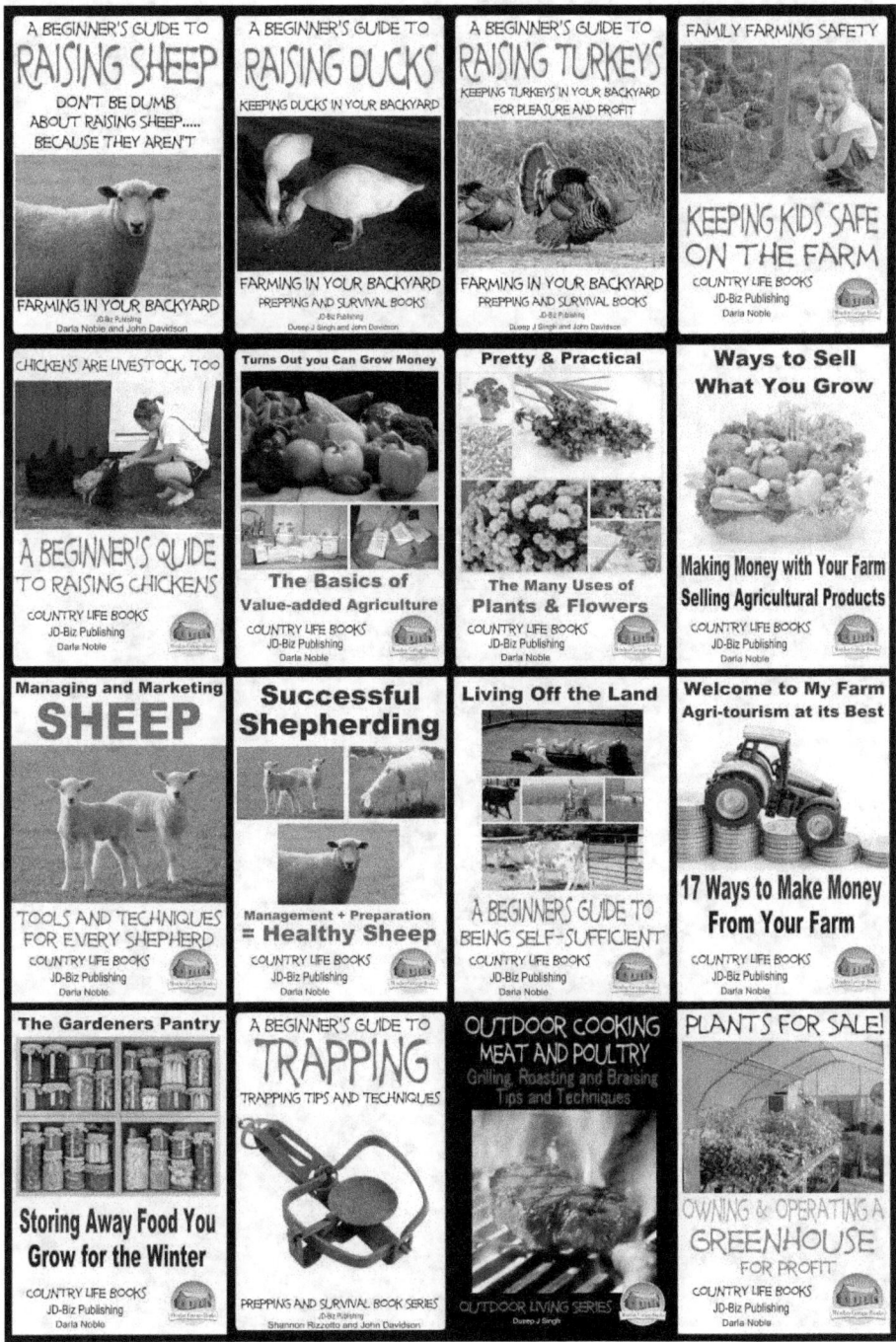

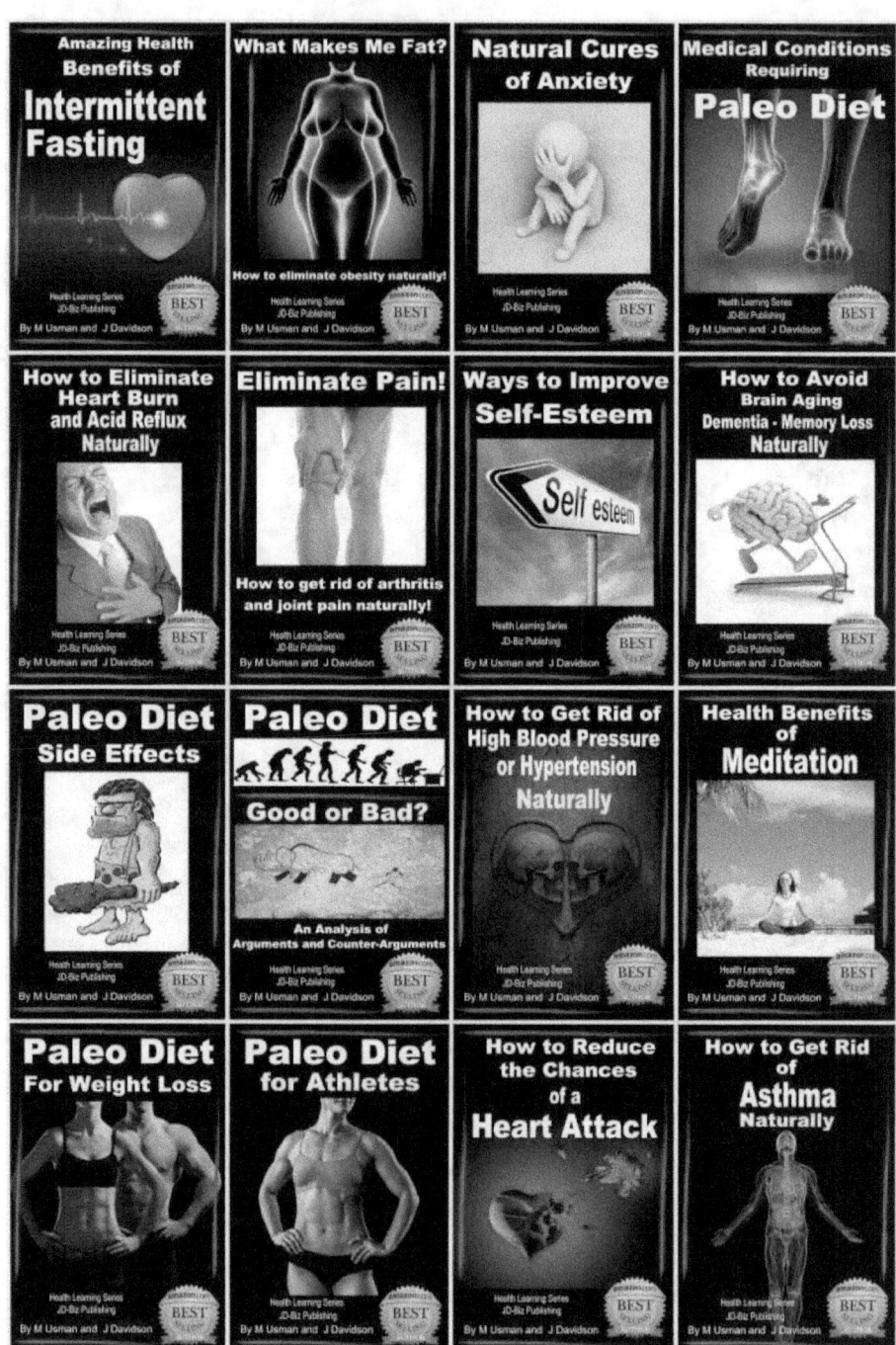

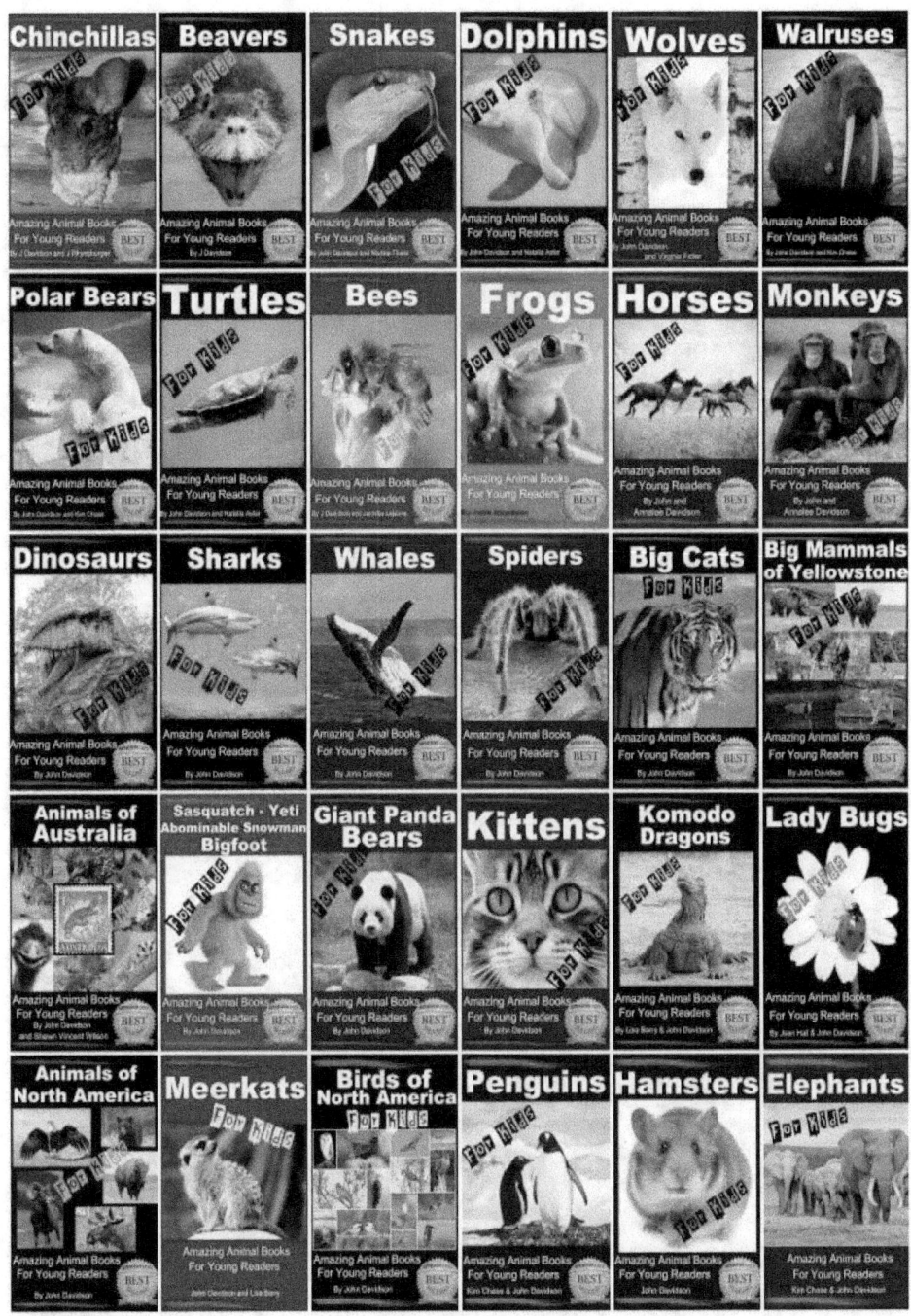

Learn To Draw Series

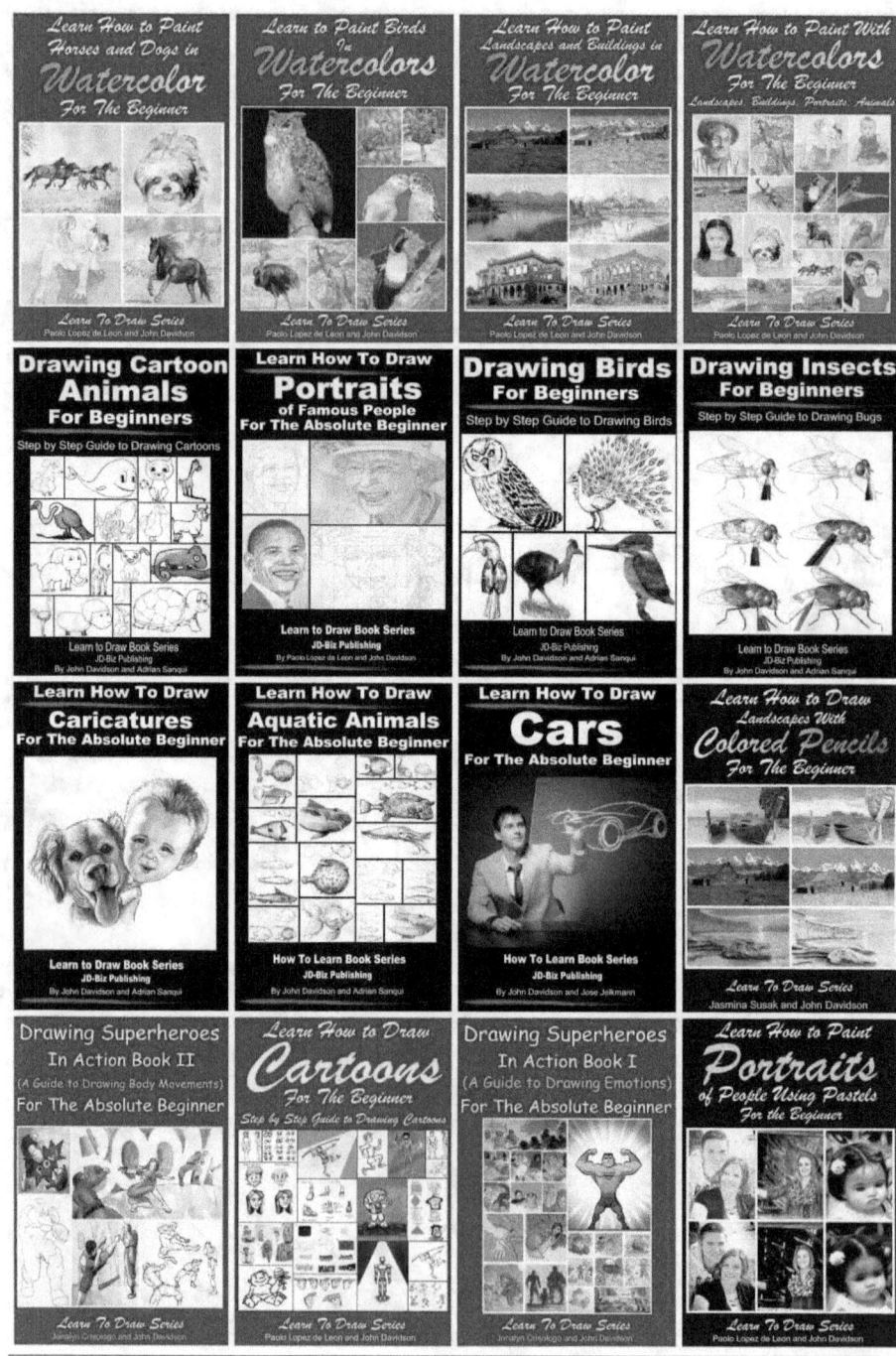

How to Build and Plan Books

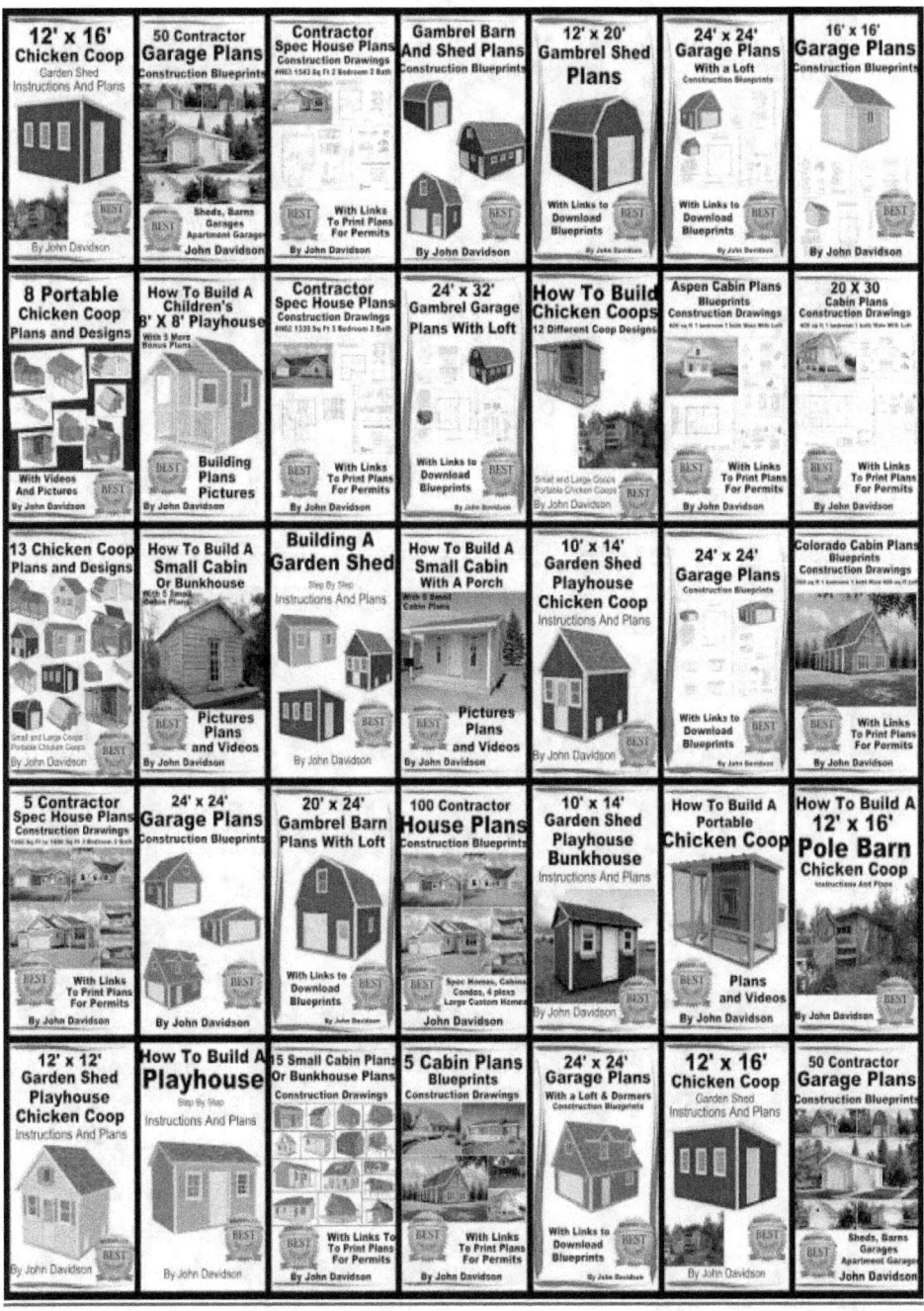

Entrepreneur Book Series

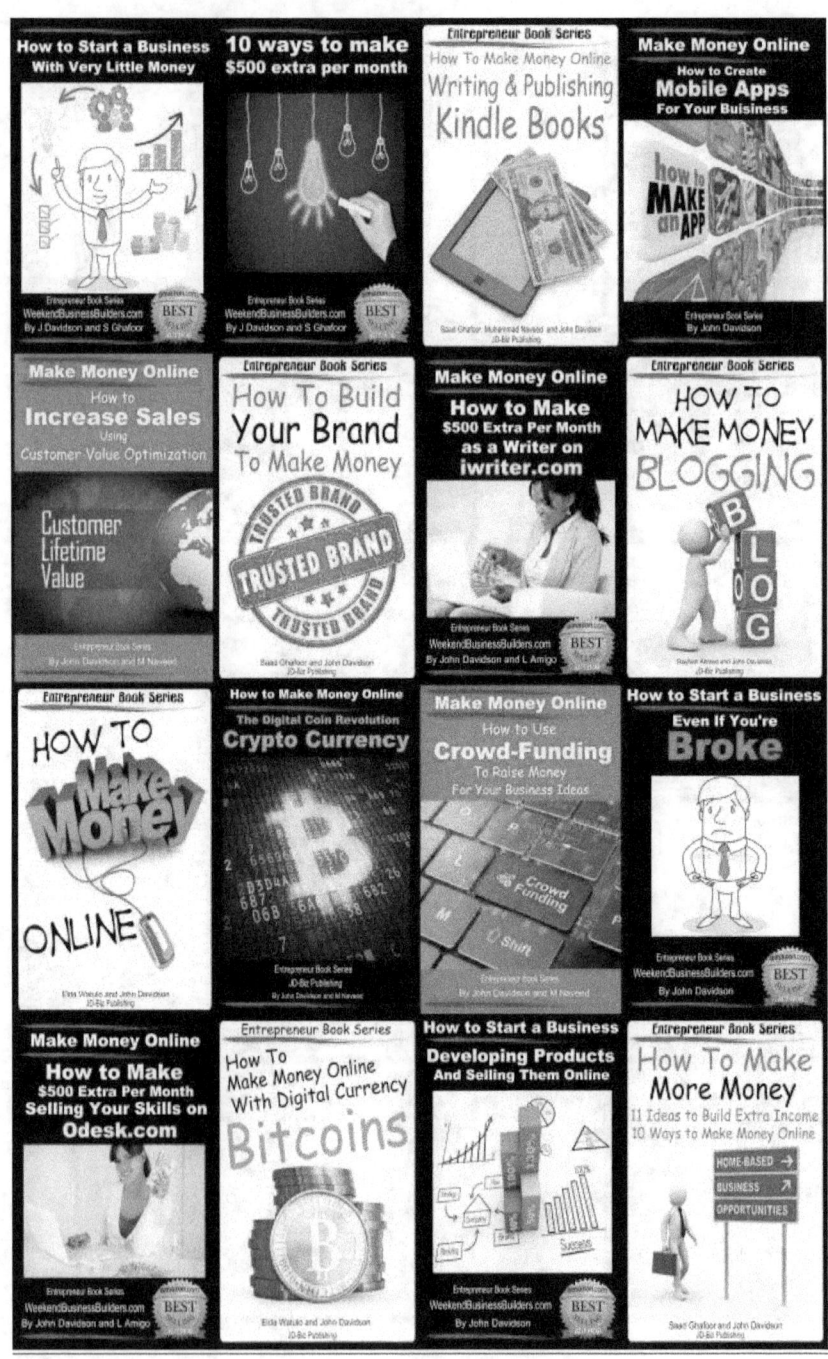

Our books are available at

1. Amazon.com

2. Barnes and Noble

3. Itunes

4. Kobo

5. Smashwords

6. Google Play Books

Publisher

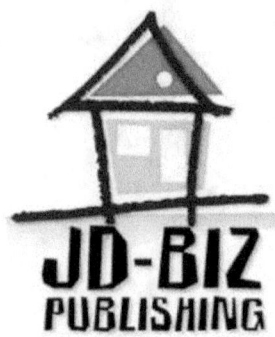

JD-Biz Corp

P O Box 374

Mendon, Utah 84325

http://www.jd-biz.com/

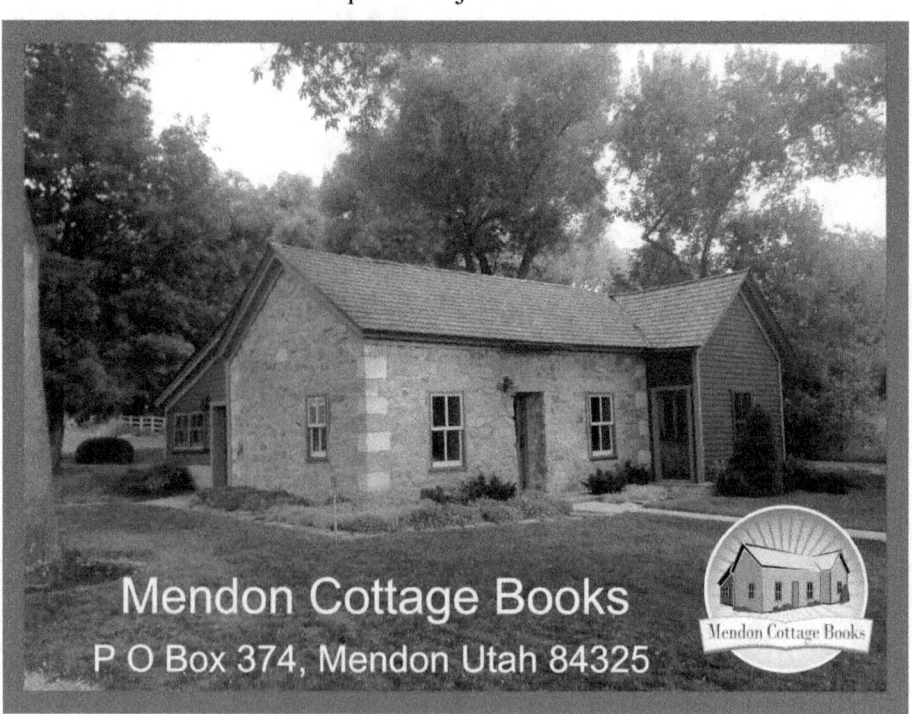

Mendon Cottage Books

P O Box 374, Mendon Utah 84325

www.ingramcontent.com/pod-product-compliance
Lightning Source LLC
Chambersburg PA
CBHW061930280526
45787CB00004B/1552

* 9 7 8 1 5 0 7 5 8 1 6 4 3 *